Plant Based Anti-Inflammatory Cookbook

Tracey Savage

Disclaimer

Please bear in mind that the information in this book is strictly educational. The data presented here is claimed to be credible and trustworthy. The author provides no implied or explicit assurance of accuracy for specific individual instances.

It is important that you consult with a skilled practitioner, such as your doctor, before initiating any diet or lifestyle changes. The information in this book should not be used in place of expert advice or professional assistance.

The author, publisher, and distributor fully disclaim any and all liability, loss, damage, or risk suffered by anybody who relies on the information in this book, whether directly or indirectly.

All intellectual property rights are intact. The content in this book should not be copied in any way, mechanically, electronically, by photocopying, or by any other means available.

CONTENTS

Introduction

In recent years, there has been a growing awareness of the profound impact that diet can have on overall health and well-being. Among the various dietary approaches gaining recognition, plant-based eating has emerged as a powerful and transformative way to promote health. This shift in dietary focus is not merely a passing trend but is backed by extensive scientific research highlighting the numerous benefits associated with plant-centric diets.

One key aspect that has captured the attention of researchers and health enthusiasts alike is the relationship between diet and inflammation. Inflammation, a natural immune response designed to protect the body, can become chronic and harmful when prolonged. This chronic inflammation has been linked to a range of health issues, including cardiovascular diseases, diabetes, and autoimmune disorders. Understanding the mechanisms of inflammation and how dietary choices can influence its regulation is pivotal for taking control of one's health.

Scientific studies have consistently demonstrated the profound impact of dietary choices on the body's inflammatory response. Certain foods, especially those rich in processed sugars, unhealthy fats, and additives, have been identified as contributors to chronic inflammation. In contrast, a plant-based diet, characterized by a rich array of fruits, vegetables, whole grains, legumes, and nuts, has been shown to possess potent anti-inflammatory properties. This link between plant-based eating and inflammation management forms the foundation of a holistic approach to health and longevity.

The benefits of adopting a plant-based, anti-inflammatory diet are extensive and multifaceted. Firstly, such a diet is naturally abundant in essential nutrients, antioxidants, and phytochemicals, all of which play crucial roles in reducing inflammation and supporting overall immune function. Additionally, plant-based diets are associated with lower levels of cholesterol and blood pressure, reducing the risk of cardiovascular diseases. Moreover, these diets are often effective in promoting weight management and reducing the incidence of obesity-related inflammation, thereby preventing a myriad of health complications.

This cookbook is crafted with the intention of harnessing the power of plant-based eating to combat inflammation and enhance well-being. Each recipe is meticulously designed to not only tantalize the taste buds but also to provide a rich array of nutrients that actively work to quell inflammation. From vibrant salads bursting with colorful vegetables to hearty grain bowls featuring a variety of whole grains and legumes, every dish is a step towards a healthier, more vibrant life. The carefully curated recipes aim to make the transition to a plant-based lifestyle seamless and enjoyable, proving that nourishing your body can be a delicious and satisfying experience.

Embarking on a plant-based journey may seem daunting at first, but with the right guidance, it can be a rewarding and transformative experience. In the following sections, we will provide practical tips and insights to help you succeed on your plant-based journey. From navigating grocery aisles to mastering plant-based cooking techniques, these tips are designed to empower you with the knowledge and skills needed to make lasting, positive changes to your dietary habits.

As you delve into the pages of this cookbook, you are not only gaining access to a collection of delectable recipes but also opening the door to a healthier, more vibrant lifestyle. The power of plant-based eating extends far beyond the confines of the kitchen; it is a journey towards enhanced well-being, vitality, and longevity. Let this cookbook be your guide as you embark on a flavorful and nourishing adventure towards a plant-powered, anti-inflammatory lifestyle.

Chapter 1: Foundations of a Plant-Based Diet

Overview of Plant-Based Eating

The journey toward embracing a plant-based diet begins with a comprehensive understanding of the principles that underpin this transformative approach to nutrition. Plant-based eating revolves around the consumption of whole, minimally processed foods derived from plant sources. This includes a diverse array of fruits, vegetables, legumes, whole grains, nuts, and seeds. The emphasis is on filling your plate with nutrient-dense, plant-derived foods that provide a broad spectrum of vitamins, minerals, antioxidants, and fiber. By centering meals on plant-based ingredients, individuals can reap the health benefits associated with reduced inflammation, improved heart health, and enhanced overall well-being.

Building a Balanced Plate

A key tenet of a successful plant-based diet is the construction of a well-balanced plate. This involves incorporating a variety of plant foods to ensure a comprehensive intake of essential nutrients. A colorful plate, featuring a mix of vegetables, fruits, whole grains, and plant-based proteins, not only adds visual appeal to meals but also ensures a diverse nutrient profile. The aim is to create meals that are not only satisfying but also nutritionally robust, providing the body with the necessary building blocks for optimal functioning.

Essential Nutrients for Inflammation Control

In the context of inflammation control, certain nutrients play a pivotal role in modulating the body's immune response. Antioxidants, for example, found abundantly in fruits and vegetables, help neutralize free radicals and reduce oxidative stress, a major contributor to chronic inflammation. Essential fatty acids, particularly omega-3s, found in flaxseeds, chia seeds, walnuts, and algae, also contribute to inflammation control. Understanding how these nutrients work synergistically to support the body in managing inflammation is crucial for crafting a plant-based diet that promotes overall health and wellness. Plant-Based Protein Sources

A common concern for those transitioning to a plant-based diet is ensuring an adequate intake of protein. Contrary to the misconception that plant-based diets lack protein, there are numerous plant sources that provide ample amounts of this essential nutrient. Legumes such as lentils, chickpeas, and black beans, along with tofu, tempeh, and edamame, are excellent plant-based protein sources. Nuts and seeds, including almonds, sunflower seeds, and chia seeds, also contribute to meeting protein requirements. Understanding how to combine these sources strategically ensures a complete and balanced amino acid profile, supporting muscle maintenance and overall bodily function.

Smart Carbohydrates and Healthy Fats

Carbohydrates and fats are crucial components of a well-rounded diet, and in a plant-based context, the focus is on selecting smart carbohydrates and healthy fats. Whole grains, such as quinoa, brown rice, and oats, provide complex carbohydrates that release energy gradually, promoting sustained satiety and stable blood sugar levels. Additionally, incorporating a variety of colorful fruits and vegetables ensures a diverse intake of carbohydrates rich in fiber and essential nutrients.

Healthy fats, predominantly derived from plant sources like avocados, nuts, seeds, and olive oil, play a crucial role in supporting various bodily functions. These fats, particularly monounsaturated and polyunsaturated fats, contribute to heart health and inflammation control. Understanding how to incorporate these healthy fats into meals enhances the nutritional profile of a plant-based diet, offering a flavorful and satisfying culinary experience.

Here, we lay the foundations for a successful journey into plant-based eating by providing a comprehensive overview of the principles, nutrient considerations, and practical tips for constructing well-balanced, nourishing meals. By embracing the richness of plant-derived foods and understanding their nutritional value, you are poised to embark on a path that not only supports inflammation control but also promotes overall health and vitality. As you delve into the subsequent chapters, the knowledge gained here will serve as a solid framework for creating delicious, plant-powered dishes that contribute to your well-being and longevity.

Breakfast

Quinoa Breakfast Bowl with Mixed Berries

- Total Time: 20 minutes
- Servings: 2

Ingredients:
- 1 cup cooked quinoa
- 1 cup mixed berries (strawberries, blueberries, raspberries)
- 1 tablespoon maple syrup
- 1/4 cup chopped nuts (almonds, walnuts)
- 1 tablespoon chia seeds
- 1/2 cup almond milk
- Fresh mint leaves for garnish

Directions:
1. In a bowl, combine cooked quinoa, mixed berries, maple syrup, chopped nuts, and chia seeds.
2. Pour almond milk over the mixture and stir well.
3. Garnish with fresh mint leaves and serve.

Nutritional Information (per serving):
- Calories: 300
- Protein: 8g
- Carbohydrates: 45g
- Fiber: 9g
- Fat: 12g

Sweet Potato and Kale Breakfast Hash

- Total Time: 25 minutes
- Servings: 2

Ingredients:

- 2 medium sweet potatoes, diced
- 2 cups kale, chopped
- 1 red onion, diced
- 2 tablespoons olive oil
- 1 teaspoon smoked paprika
- Salt and pepper to taste
- 1 avocado, sliced (for garnish)

Directions:

1. In a skillet, heat olive oil over medium heat. Add diced sweet potatoes and cook until golden brown.
2. Add red onion, kale, smoked paprika, salt, and pepper. Cook until kale is wilted.
3. Serve hot, garnished with sliced avocado.

Nutritional Information (per serving):

- Calories: 320
- Protein: 5g
- Carbohydrates: 45g
- Fiber: 10g
- Fat: 15g

Chia Seed Pudding with Almond Milk and Berries

- Total Time: 4 hours (includes chilling time)
- Servings: 2

Ingredients:
- 1/4 cup chia seeds
- 1 cup almond milk
- 1 tablespoon maple syrup
- 1/2 teaspoon vanilla extract
- Mixed berries for topping

Directions:
1. In a bowl, whisk together chia seeds, almond milk, maple syrup, and vanilla extract.
2. Refrigerate for at least 4 hours or overnight.
3. Top with mixed berries before serving.

Nutritional Information (per serving):
- Calories: 180
- Protein: 5g
- Carbohydrates: 20g
- Fiber: 12g
- Fat: 9g

Turmeric Oatmeal with Walnuts and Mango

- Total Time: 15 minutes
- Servings: 2

Ingredients:
- 1 cup rolled oats

- 2 cups water
- 1/2 teaspoon ground turmeric
- 1/4 cup chopped walnuts
- 1 ripe mango, diced
- 1 tablespoon maple syrup
- Pinch of black pepper

Directions:

1. Cook rolled oats in water with ground turmeric until creamy.
2. Top with chopped walnuts, diced mango, maple syrup, and a pinch of black pepper.

Nutritional Information (per serving):

- Calories: 320
- Protein: 8g
- Carbohydrates: 55g
- Fiber: 8g
- Fat: 10g

Spinach and Mushroom Vegan Omelette

- Total Time: 20 minutes
- Servings: 2

Ingredients:

- 1 cup chickpea flour
- 1 1/4 cups water
- 1 tablespoon nutritional yeast
- 1/2 teaspoon turmeric powder
- Salt and pepper to taste
- 1 cup spinach, chopped
- 1/2 cup mushrooms, sliced

- 1/4 cup red bell pepper, diced
- 1 tablespoon olive oil

Directions:
1. In a bowl, whisk chickpea flour, water, nutritional yeast, turmeric, salt, and pepper.
2. In a skillet, sauté spinach, mushrooms, and red bell pepper in olive oil.
3. Pour chickpea flour mixture over the veggies and cook until set. Fold the omelette and serve.

Nutritional Information (per serving):
- Calories: 220
- Protein: 12g
- Carbohydrates: 25g
- Fiber: 6g
- Fat: 10g

Blueberry Banana Smoothie Bowl

- Total Time: 10 minutes
- Servings: 2

Ingredients:
- 2 frozen bananas
- 1 cup blueberries
- 1/2 cup almond milk
- 2 tablespoons chia seeds
- Toppings: granola, sliced bananas, shredded coconut

Directions:
1. Blend frozen bananas, blueberries, and almond milk until smooth.

2. Pour into bowls and top with chia seeds, granola, sliced bananas, and shredded coconut.

Nutritional Information (per serving):
- Calories: 250
- Protein: 5g
- Carbohydrates: 45g
- Fiber: 10g
- Fat: 7g

Avocado Toast with Cherry Tomatoes and Microgreens

- Total Time: 10 minutes
- Servings: 2

Ingredients:
- 2 slices whole grain bread, toasted
- 1 ripe avocado, mashed
- 1 cup cherry tomatoes, halved
- Microgreens for garnish
- Salt and pepper to taste
- Optional: red pepper flakes for a kick

Directions:
1. Spread mashed avocado on toasted bread slices.
2. Top with cherry tomatoes, microgreens, salt, pepper, and optional red pepper flakes.

Nutritional Information (per serving):
- Calories: 220
- Protein: 5g
- Carbohydrates: 30g
- Fiber: 10g
- Fat: 10g

Vegan Pancakes with Maple Syrup and Pecans

- **Total Time:** 20 minutes
- **Servings:** 2

Ingredients:
- 1 cup all-purpose flour
- 1 tablespoon sugar
- 1 tablespoon baking powder
- 1 cup almond milk
- 2 tablespoons coconut oil (melted)
- 1 teaspoon vanilla extract
- Maple syrup and pecans for topping

Directions:
1. In a bowl, whisk together flour, sugar, and baking powder.
2. Add almond milk, melted coconut oil, and vanilla extract. Mix until just combined.
3. Heat a griddle or skillet over medium heat. Pour 1/4 cup of batter for each pancake.
4. Cook until bubbles form on the surface, then flip and cook until golden brown.
5. Serve with maple syrup and sprinkle with pecans.

Nutritional Information (per serving):
- **Calories:** 350
- **Protein:** 8g
- **Carbohydrates:** 45g
- **Fiber:** 4g
- **Fat:** 15g

Mango Turmeric Smoothie

- **Total Time:** 10 minutes
- **Servings:** 1

Ingredients:

- 1 cup frozen mango chunks
- 1/2 banana
- 1/2 teaspoon turmeric powder
- 1 cup coconut water
- 1 tablespoon chia seeds
- Ice cubes (optional)

Directions:

1. In a blender, combine frozen mango chunks, banana, turmeric powder, coconut water, and chia seeds.
2. Blend until smooth.
3. Add ice cubes if desired and blend again.
4. Pour into a glass and enjoy.

Nutritional Information (per serving):

- **Calories:** 280
- **Protein:** 5g
- **Carbohydrates:** 55g
- **Fiber:** 10g
- **Fat:** 7g

Almond Butter and Banana Breakfast Wrap

- **Total Time:** 10 minutes
- **Servings:** 1

Ingredients:

- 1 whole grain tortilla
- 2 tablespoons almond butter
- 1 banana, sliced
- 1 teaspoon chia seeds
- Drizzle of honey (optional)

Directions:

1. Spread almond butter on the whole grain tortilla.
2. Place banana slices on one side and sprinkle with chia seeds.
3. Drizzle with honey if desired.
4. Fold the tortilla, cut in half, and serve.

Nutritional Information (per serving):

- **Calories:** 380
- **Protein:** 8g
- **Carbohydrates:** 45g
- **Fiber:** 8g
- **Fat:** 20g

Vegan Breakfast Burrito with Black Beans and Salsa

- **Total Time:** 15 minutes
- **Servings:** 2

Ingredients:

- 1 cup black beans (canned, drained, and rinsed)
- 1/2 cup salsa
- 1 avocado, sliced
- 2 whole grain tortillas
- Fresh cilantro for garnish
- Salt and pepper to taste

Directions:

1. In a bowl, mix black beans with salsa.
2. Warm tortillas and spoon the bean mixture onto each.
3. Top with avocado slices, cilantro, salt, and pepper.
4. Roll into burritos and serve.

Nutritional Information (per serving):

- **Calories:** 420
- **Protein:** 12g
- **Carbohydrates:** 60g
- **Fiber:** 15g
- **Fat:** 18g

Green Tea Infused Overnight Oats

- **Total Time:** 8 hours (overnight)
- **Servings:** 1

Ingredients:
- 1/2 cup rolled oats
- 1/2 cup green tea (cooled)
- 1/2 cup almond milk
- 1 tablespoon maple syrup
- 1/2 teaspoon matcha powder
- Sliced kiwi for topping

Directions:
1. In a jar, combine rolled oats, green tea, almond milk, maple syrup, and matcha powder.
2. Stir well, cover, and refrigerate overnight.
3. In the morning, top with sliced kiwi and enjoy.

Nutritional Information (per serving):
- **Calories:** 280
- **Protein:** 7g
- **Carbohydrates:** 45g
- **Fiber:** 8g
- **Fat:** 8g

Chickpea Flour Scramble with Spinach and Tomatoes

- **Total Time:** 15 minutes
- **Servings:** 2

Ingredients:
- 1 cup chickpea flour

- 1 1/4 cups water
- 1 tablespoon nutritional yeast
- 1/2 teaspoon turmeric powder
- Salt and pepper to taste
- 1 cup spinach, chopped
- 1/2 cup cherry tomatoes, halved
- 1 tablespoon olive oil

Directions:

1. In a bowl, whisk chickpea flour, water, nutritional yeast, turmeric, salt, and pepper.
2. In a skillet, sauté spinach and cherry tomatoes in olive oil.
3. Pour chickpea flour mixture over the veggies and cook until set.
4. Serve hot.

Nutritional Information (per serving):

- **Calories:** 220
- **Protein:** 10g
- **Carbohydrates:** 25g
- **Fiber:** 6g
- **Fat:** 10g

Berry and Spinach Smoothie

- **Total Time:** 10 minutes
- **Servings:** 1

Ingredients:

- 1 cup mixed berries (strawberries, blueberries, raspberries)
- 1/2 cup spinach
- 1/2 banana

- 1/2 cup almond milk
- 1 tablespoon flaxseeds
- Ice cubes (optional)

Directions:
1. In a blender, combine mixed berries, spinach, banana, almond milk, and flaxseeds.
2. Blend until smooth.
3. Add ice cubes if desired and blend again.
4. Pour into a glass and enjoy.

Nutritional Information (per serving):
- **Calories:** 210
- **Protein:** 5g
- **Carbohydrates:** 35g
- **Fiber:** 8g
- **Fat:** 7g

Vegan French Toast with Cinnamon and Maple Syrup

- **Total Time:** 15 minutes
- **Servings:** 2

Ingredients:
- 4 slices whole grain bread
- 1/2 cup almond milk
- 2 tablespoons chickpea flour
- 1 teaspoon cinnamon
- 1 teaspoon vanilla extract
- Maple syrup for drizzling
- Fresh berries for topping

Directions:
1. In a bowl, whisk together almond milk, chickpea flour, cinnamon, and vanilla extract.
2. Dip each bread slice into the mixture, ensuring it's coated on both sides.
3. Cook on a griddle or skillet until golden brown on both sides.
4. Drizzle with maple syrup and top with fresh berries.

Nutritional Information (per serving):
- **Calories:** 250
- **Protein:** 7g
- **Carbohydrates:** 45g
- **Fiber:** 8g
- **Fat:** 6g

Lunch

Quinoa and Black Bean Stuffed Peppers

- **Total Time:** 45 minutes
- **Servings:** 4

Ingredients:
- 4 large bell peppers, halved and seeds removed
- 1 cup quinoa, cooked
- 1 can black beans, drained and rinsed
- 1 cup corn kernels
- 1 cup diced tomatoes
- 1 teaspoon cumin
- 1 teaspoon chili powder
- Salt and pepper to taste
- Salsa and avocado for topping

Directions:
1. Preheat the oven to 375°F (190°C).
2. In a bowl, mix cooked quinoa, black beans, corn, diced tomatoes, cumin, chili powder, salt, and pepper.
3. Stuff each pepper half with the quinoa mixture.
4. Bake for 25-30 minutes or until peppers are tender.
5. Top with salsa and sliced avocado before serving.

Nutritional Information (per serving):
- **Calories:** 350
- **Protein:** 12g
- **Carbohydrates:** 60g
- **Fiber:** 12g
- **Fat:** 8g

Lentil and Vegetable Soup with Turmeric

- **Total Time:** 40 minutes
- **Servings:** 6

Ingredients:
- 1 cup dried green lentils, rinsed
- 1 onion, diced
- 2 carrots, diced
- 2 celery stalks, diced
- 3 cloves garlic, minced
- 1 teaspoon turmeric powder
- 1 teaspoon cumin
- 6 cups vegetable broth
- Salt and pepper to taste
- Fresh parsley for garnish

Directions:
1. In a large pot, sauté onion, carrots, celery, and garlic until softened.
2. Add turmeric, cumin, lentils, and vegetable broth. Bring to a boil.
3. Reduce heat and simmer until lentils are tender, about 25 minutes.
4. Season with salt and pepper. Garnish with fresh parsley before serving.

Nutritional Information (per serving):
- **Calories:** 220
- **Protein:** 14g
- **Carbohydrates:** 35g
- **Fiber:** 10g
- **Fat:** 2g

Grilled Portobello Mushroom Wraps with Hummus

- **Total Time:** 20 minutes
- **Servings:** 2

Ingredients:
- 4 large portobello mushrooms, cleaned and sliced
- 2 whole wheat wraps
- 1 cup cherry tomatoes, halved
- 1 cucumber, sliced
- 1/2 cup hummus
- Fresh basil leaves for garnish
- Salt and pepper to taste

Directions:
1. Grill portobello mushrooms until tender, about 5 minutes per side.
2. Spread hummus on each wrap.
3. Fill wraps with grilled mushrooms, cherry tomatoes, and cucumber slices.
4. Season with salt and pepper, and garnish with fresh basil.

Nutritional Information (per serving):
- **Calories:** 300
- **Protein:** 12g
- **Carbohydrates:** 45g
- **Fiber:** 10g
- **Fat:** 10g

Vegan Caesar Salad with Chickpea Croutons

- **Total Time:** 15 minutes
- **Servings:** 4

Ingredients:

- 1 head romaine lettuce, chopped
- 1 cup cherry tomatoes, halved
- 1/2 cup vegan Caesar dressing
- 1/4 cup nutritional yeast
- 1 can chickpeas, drained and rinsed
- 1 teaspoon garlic powder
- Salt and pepper to taste
- Lemon wedges for serving

Directions:

1. Preheat the oven to 400°F (200°C).
2. Toss chickpeas with garlic powder, salt, and pepper. Roast for 20 minutes until crispy.
3. In a large bowl, combine chopped romaine, cherry tomatoes, vegan Caesar dressing, and nutritional yeast.
4. Top with chickpea croutons and serve with lemon wedges.

Nutritional Information (per serving):

- **Calories:** 250
- **Protein:** 10g
- **Carbohydrates:** 30g
- **Fiber:** 10g
- **Fat:** 12g

Roasted Vegetable Buddha Bowl

- **Total Time:** 30 minutes
- **Servings:** 2

Ingredients:
- 1 cup quinoa, cooked
- 1 sweet potato, diced
- 1 zucchini, sliced
- 1 cup cherry tomatoes
- 1 cup broccoli florets
- 2 tablespoons olive oil
- 1 teaspoon cumin
- 1 teaspoon paprika
- Salt and pepper to taste
- Tahini dressing for drizzling

Directions:
1. Preheat the oven to 425°F (220°C).
2. Toss sweet potato, zucchini, cherry tomatoes, and broccoli with olive oil, cumin, paprika, salt, and pepper.
3. Roast for 20-25 minutes until vegetables are tender.
4. Assemble bowls with cooked quinoa and roasted vegetables. Drizzle with tahini dressing.

Nutritional Information (per serving):
- **Calories:** 380
- **Protein:** 10g
- **Carbohydrates:** 60g
- **Fiber:** 10g
- **Fat:** 12g

Spinach and Lentil Salad with Lemon-Tahini Dressing

- **Total Time:** 25 minutes
- **Servings:** 4

Ingredients:
- 2 cups cooked lentils
- 4 cups fresh spinach
- 1 cucumber, diced
- 1 cup cherry tomatoes, halved
- 1/4 cup red onion, finely chopped
- 1/3 cup sunflower seeds

Lemon-Tahini Dressing:
- 3 tablespoons tahini
- 2 tablespoons lemon juice
- 1 tablespoon olive oil
- 1 tablespoon maple syrup
- Salt and pepper to taste

Directions:
1. In a large bowl, combine cooked lentils, fresh spinach, cucumber, cherry tomatoes, red onion, and sunflower seeds.
2. In a small bowl, whisk together tahini, lemon juice, olive oil, maple syrup, salt, and pepper to create the dressing.
3. Pour the dressing over the salad and toss to combine.

Nutritional Information (per serving):
- **Calories:** 320
- **Protein:** 15g
- **Carbohydrates:** 40g

- **Fiber:** 12g
- **Fat:** 14g

Mediterranean Chickpea Salad

- **Total Time:** 15 minutes
- **Servings:** 4

Ingredients:
- 2 cans chickpeas, drained and rinsed
- 1 cucumber, diced
- 1 cup cherry tomatoes, halved
- 1/2 cup red onion, finely chopped
- 1/3 cup Kalamata olives, sliced
- 1/4 cup fresh parsley, chopped
- Feta cheese (optional)

Greek dressing:
- 1/4 cup olive oil
- 2 tablespoons red wine vinegar
- 1 teaspoon dried oregano
- Salt and pepper to taste

Directions:
1. In a large bowl, combine chickpeas, cucumber, cherry tomatoes, red onion, olives, and parsley.
2. In a small bowl, whisk together olive oil, red wine vinegar, dried oregano, salt, and pepper to make the dressing.
3. Pour the dressing over the salad and toss to coat. Top with feta if desired.

Nutritional Information (per serving):
- **Calories:** 320
- **Protein:** 12g

- **Carbohydrates:** 40g
- **Fiber:** 10g
- **Fat:** 14g

Sweet Potato and Kale Salad with Avocado

- **Total Time:** 30 minutes
- **Servings:** 2

Ingredients:
- 2 sweet potatoes, cubed
- 1 bunch kale, stems removed and chopped
- 1 avocado, sliced
- 1/4 cup pumpkin seeds
- 2 tablespoons olive oil
- 1 tablespoon balsamic vinegar
- Salt and pepper to taste

Directions:
1. Preheat the oven to 400°F (200°C).
2. Toss sweet potatoes in olive oil, salt, and pepper. Roast for 20 minutes until tender.
3. Massage kale with balsamic vinegar until slightly wilted.
4. Assemble the salad with roasted sweet potatoes, kale, avocado slices, and pumpkin seeds.

Nutritional Information (per serving):
- **Calories:** 350
- **Protein:** 8g
- **Carbohydrates:** 45g
- **Fiber:** 12g
- **Fat:** 18g

Vegan BBQ Jackfruit Tacos

- **Total Time:** 25 minutes
- **Servings:** 4

Ingredients:
- 2 cans young jackfruit in brine, drained and shredded
- 1 cup BBQ sauce
- 8 small corn tortillas
- 1 cup shredded cabbage
- 1/2 cup red onion, thinly sliced
- 1/4 cup cilantro, chopped
- Lime wedges for serving

Directions:
1. In a pan, sauté shredded jackfruit in BBQ sauce until heated through.
2. Warm corn tortillas.
3. Assemble tacos with BBQ jackfruit, shredded cabbage, red onion, and cilantro.
4. Serve with lime wedges.

Nutritional Information (per serving):
- **Calories:** 280
- **Protein:** 6g
- **Carbohydrates:** 50g
- **Fiber:** 8g
- **Fat:** 7g

Broccoli and Quinoa Patties

- **Total Time:** 35 minutes
- **Servings:** 3

Ingredients:
- 1 cup cooked quinoa
- 1 cup broccoli, finely chopped
- 1/4 cup red bell pepper, diced
- 2 green onions, sliced
- 1/4 cup nutritional yeast
- 2 tablespoons flaxseed meal mixed with 5 tablespoons water (flax egg)
- 1 teaspoon garlic powder
- Salt and pepper to taste
- 2 tablespoons olive oil for cooking

Directions:
1. In a bowl, mix quinoa, broccoli, red bell pepper, green onions, nutritional yeast, flax egg, garlic powder, salt, and pepper.
2. Form the mixture into patties.
3. Heat olive oil in a pan and cook patties until golden brown on each side.

Nutritional Information (per serving):
- **Calories:** 220
- **Protein:** 10g
- **Carbohydrates:** 30g
- **Fiber:** 8g
- **Fat:** 8g

Vegan Chickpea and Vegetable Stir-Fry

- **Total Time:** 20 minutes
- **Servings:** 2

Ingredients:
- 1 can chickpeas, drained and rinsed
- 2 cups mixed vegetables (broccoli, bell peppers, snap peas)
- 1 cup snow peas
- 2 tablespoons soy sauce
- 1 tablespoon sesame oil
- 1 teaspoon ginger, minced
- 1 teaspoon garlic, minced
- 1 tablespoon sesame seeds for garnish

Directions:
1. In a wok or skillet, sauté chickpeas and mixed vegetables in sesame oil until vegetables are tender.
2. Add snow peas, soy sauce, ginger, and garlic. Stir-fry for an additional 3-5 minutes.
3. Garnish with sesame seeds and serve over rice or quinoa.

Nutritional Information (per serving):
- **Calories:** 320
- **Protein:** 12g
- **Carbohydrates:** 45g
- **Fiber:** 12g
- **Fat:** 10g

Butternut Squash and Coconut Curry Soup

- **Total Time:** 45 minutes
- **Servings:** 4

Ingredients:

- 1 butternut squash, peeled and diced
- 1 can coconut milk
- 1 onion, diced
- 2 cloves garlic, minced
- 1 tablespoon curry powder
- 4 cups vegetable broth
- 2 tablespoons olive oil
- Salt and pepper to taste
- Fresh cilantro for garnish

Directions:

1. In a pot, sauté onion and garlic in olive oil until softened.
2. Add diced butternut squash and curry powder. Cook for 5 minutes.
3. Pour in coconut milk and vegetable broth. Simmer until squash is tender.
4. Blend the soup until smooth. Season with salt and pepper.
5. Garnish with fresh cilantro before serving.

Nutritional Information (per serving):

- **Calories:** 280
- **Protein:** 4g
- **Carbohydrates:** 30g
- **Fiber:** 8g
- **Fat:** 18g

Brown Rice and Black Bean Burrito Bowl

- **Total Time:** 30 minutes
- **Servings:** 2

Ingredients:
- 1 cup cooked brown rice
- 1 can black beans, drained and rinsed
- 1 cup corn kernels
- 1 avocado, sliced
- 1/2 cup salsa
- 1/4 cup fresh cilantro, chopped
- Lime wedges for serving

Directions:
1. In bowls, layer brown rice, black beans, corn, avocado slices, and salsa.
2. Top with fresh cilantro and serve with lime wedges.

Nutritional Information (per serving):
- **Calories:** 380
- **Protein:** 10g
- **Carbohydrates:** 60g
- **Fiber:** 12g
- **Fat:** 10g

Zucchini Noodles with Pesto and Cherry Tomatoes

- **Total Time:** 15 minutes
- **Servings:** 2

Ingredients:
- 2 large zucchinis, spiralized
- 1 cup cherry tomatoes, halved
- 1/4 cup pine nuts
- 1/2 cup fresh basil leaves
- 2 tablespoons nutritional yeast
- 2 tablespoons olive oil
- 1 clove garlic, minced
- Salt and pepper to taste

Directions:
1. In a blender, combine basil, pine nuts, nutritional yeast, olive oil, garlic, salt, and pepper. Blend until smooth.
2. Toss zucchini noodles with pesto and cherry tomatoes.
3. Serve immediately.

Nutritional Information (per serving):
- **Calories:** 220
- **Protein:** 6g
- **Carbohydrates:** 15g
- **Fiber:** 5g
- **Fat:** 18g

Sweet Potato and Chickpea Buddha Bowl

- **Total Time:** 40 minutes
- **Servings:** 2

Ingredients:
- 1 large sweet potato, cubed
- 1 can chickpeas, drained and rinsed
- 1 tablespoon olive oil
- 1 teaspoon smoked paprika
- 2 cups quinoa, cooked
- 1 avocado, sliced
- 1/4 cup tahini
- Fresh parsley for garnish
- Salt and pepper to taste

Directions:
1. Preheat the oven to 400°F (200°C).
2. Toss sweet potato and chickpeas in olive oil, smoked paprika, salt, and pepper. Roast for 25-30 minutes until golden.
3. Assemble bowls with cooked quinoa, roasted sweet potato and chickpeas, avocado slices, and a drizzle of tahini.
4. Garnish with fresh parsley.

Nutritional Information (per serving):
- **Calories:** 420
- **Protein:** 14g
- **Carbohydrates:** 60g
- **Fiber:** 12g
- **Fat:** 16g

Dinner

Eggplant and Lentil Moussaka

- **Total Time:** 1 hour 30 minutes
- **Servings:** 6

Ingredients:
- 2 large eggplants, sliced
- 1 cup dry green lentils, cooked
- 1 onion, finely chopped
- 3 cloves garlic, minced
- 1 can crushed tomatoes
- 1 teaspoon dried oregano
- 1 teaspoon ground cinnamon
- 1/2 teaspoon ground nutmeg
- 2 tablespoons olive oil
- Salt and pepper to taste
- Vegan béchamel sauce (store-bought or homemade)

Directions:
1. Preheat the oven to 375°F (190°C).
2. In a pan, sauté onion and garlic in olive oil until softened.
3. Add cooked lentils, crushed tomatoes, oregano, cinnamon, nutmeg, salt, and pepper. Simmer for 15 minutes.
4. In a separate pan, grill eggplant slices until lightly browned.
5. In a baking dish, layer grilled eggplant and lentil mixture. Repeat layers.
6. Top with vegan béchamel sauce.
7. Bake for 40-45 minutes until golden and bubbly.

Nutritional Information (per serving):

- **Calories:** 350
- **Protein:** 14g
- **Carbohydrates:** 45g
- **Fiber:** 12g
- **Fat:** 15g

Vegan Mushroom and Spinach Lasagna

- **Total Time:** 1 hour
- **Servings:** 8

Ingredients:

- 9 lasagna noodles, cooked
- 2 cups sliced mushrooms
- 4 cups fresh spinach
- 1 onion, diced
- 3 cloves garlic, minced
- 1 can crushed tomatoes
- 1 teaspoon dried basil
- 1 teaspoon dried oregano
- 2 cups vegan ricotta cheese
- 1 cup vegan mozzarella cheese, shredded
- Salt and pepper to taste
- Olive oil for sautéing

Directions:

1. Preheat the oven to 375°F (190°C).
2. In a pan, sauté onion and garlic in olive oil until softened.
3. Add mushrooms and spinach, cook until wilted.
4. Stir in crushed tomatoes, basil, oregano, salt, and pepper. Simmer for 15 minutes.

5. In a baking dish, layer lasagna noodles, mushroom-spinach mixture, vegan ricotta, and vegan mozzarella. Repeat layers.
6. Bake for 30-35 minutes until bubbly and golden.

Nutritional Information (per serving):
- **Calories:** 420
- **Protein:** 15g
- **Carbohydrates:** 50g
- **Fiber:** 8g
- **Fat:** 18g

Spaghetti Squash Primavera with Vegan Pesto

- **Total Time:** 40 minutes
- **Servings:** 4

Ingredients:
- 1 large spaghetti squash, halved and seeds removed
- 2 cups cherry tomatoes, halved
- 1 cup broccoli florets
- 1 cup baby carrots, sliced
- 1/2 cup vegan pesto
- 2 tablespoons olive oil
- Salt and pepper to taste
- Vegan Parmesan for garnish

Directions:
1. Preheat the oven to 400°F (200°C).
2. Rub spaghetti squash halves with olive oil, salt, and pepper. Roast for 30 minutes.
3. In a pan, sauté cherry tomatoes, broccoli, and carrots until tender.

4. Use a fork to shred the spaghetti squash into "noodles."
5. Toss the vegetable mixture with spaghetti squash and vegan pesto.
6. Garnish with vegan Parmesan before serving.

Nutritional Information (per serving):
- **Calories:** 280
- **Protein:** 6g
- **Carbohydrates:** 35g
- **Fiber:** 10g
- **Fat:** 15g

Chickpea and Vegetable Coconut Curry

- **Total Time:** 45 minutes
- **Servings:** 4

Ingredients:
- 1 can chickpeas, drained and rinsed
- 1 cup broccoli florets
- 1 red bell pepper, sliced
- 1 carrot, sliced
- 1 can coconut milk
- 2 tablespoons red curry paste
- 1 tablespoon soy sauce
- 1 tablespoon maple syrup
- 1 tablespoon vegetable oil
- Fresh cilantro for garnish
- Cooked basmati rice for serving

Directions:

1. In a pan, sauté broccoli, red bell pepper, and carrot in vegetable oil until slightly softened.
2. Add chickpeas, coconut milk, red curry paste, soy sauce, and maple syrup. Simmer for 15-20 minutes.
3. Serve over cooked basmati rice and garnish with fresh cilantro.

Nutritional Information (per serving):
- **Calories:** 380
- **Protein:** 10g
- **Carbohydrates:** 45g
- **Fiber:** 12g
- **Fat:** 18g

Stuffed Acorn Squash with Quinoa and Cranberries

- **Total Time:** 50 minutes
- **Servings:** 4

Ingredients:
- 2 acorn squashes, halved and seeds removed
- 1 cup quinoa, cooked
- 1/2 cup dried cranberries
- 1/2 cup pecans, chopped
- 2 tablespoons maple syrup
- 1 teaspoon cinnamon
- Olive oil for brushing
- Salt to taste

Directions:

1. Preheat the oven to 400°F (200°C).

2. Brush the cut sides of acorn squash with olive oil and sprinkle with salt. Roast for 30 minutes.
3. In a bowl, mix cooked quinoa, dried cranberries, pecans, maple syrup, and cinnamon.
4. Fill each acorn squash half with the quinoa mixture.
5. Bake for an additional 15-20 minutes until squash is tender.

Nutritional Information (per serving):
- **Calories:** 320
- **Protein:** 8g
- **Carbohydrates:** 55g
- **Fiber:** 8g
- **Fat:** 10g

Vegan Lentil Loaf with Tomato Glaze

- **Total Time:** 1 hour 15 minutes
- **Servings:** 6

Ingredients:
- 2 cups cooked green lentils
- 1 onion, finely chopped
- 2 carrots, grated
- 2 cloves garlic, minced
- 1 cup rolled oats
- 1/2 cup tomato sauce
- 1/4 cup soy sauce
- 1/4 cup nutritional yeast
- 1 teaspoon dried thyme
- 1 teaspoon dried rosemary
- Salt and pepper to taste

- Tomato glaze: 1/2 cup tomato sauce mixed with 2 tablespoons maple syrup

Directions:
1. Preheat the oven to 375°F (190°C).
2. In a bowl, combine cooked lentils, chopped onion, grated carrots, minced garlic, rolled oats, tomato sauce, soy sauce, nutritional yeast, thyme, rosemary, salt, and pepper.
3. Press the mixture into a loaf pan.
4. Bake for 45 minutes, then brush with the tomato glaze.
5. Bake for an additional 15-20 minutes until firm.

Nutritional Information (per serving):
- **Calories:** 280
- **Protein:** 14g
- **Carbohydrates:** 45g
- **Fiber:** 10g
- **Fat:** 6g

Roasted Brussels Sprouts and Cauliflower Tacos

- **Total Time:** 30 minutes
- **Servings:** 4

Ingredients:
- 2 cups Brussels sprouts, halved
- 2 cups cauliflower florets
- 2 tablespoons olive oil
- 1 teaspoon cumin
- 1 teaspoon smoked paprika
- 1/2 teaspoon garlic powder

- 1/2 teaspoon onion powder
- 8 small corn tortillas
- 1 cup red cabbage, shredded
- 1/2 cup vegan chipotle mayo
- Lime wedges for serving

Directions:

1. Preheat the oven to 425°F (220°C).
2. Toss Brussels sprouts and cauliflower with olive oil, cumin, smoked paprika, garlic powder, and onion powder.
3. Roast for 20 minutes until vegetables are crispy.
4. Warm corn tortillas.
5. Assemble tacos with roasted vegetables, shredded red cabbage, and a drizzle of vegan chipotle mayo.
6. Serve with lime wedges.

Nutritional Information (per serving):

- **Calories:** 320
- **Protein:** 8g
- **Carbohydrates:** 40g
- **Fiber:** 10g
- **Fat:** 15g

Cabbage and Lentil Soup

- **Total Time:** 45 minutes
- **Servings:** 6

Ingredients:

- 1 cup green or brown lentils, rinsed
- 1 small cabbage, shredded
- 2 carrots, diced
- 1 onion, chopped

- 3 cloves garlic, minced
- 1 can diced tomatoes
- 6 cups vegetable broth
- 1 teaspoon cumin
- 1 teaspoon paprika
- Salt and pepper to taste
- Fresh parsley for garnish

Directions:

1. In a large pot, sauté onions and garlic until softened.
2. Add lentils, cabbage, carrots, diced tomatoes, vegetable broth, cumin, paprika, salt, and pepper.
3. Bring to a boil, then simmer for 30 minutes.
4. Garnish with fresh parsley before serving.

Nutritional Information (per serving):

- **Calories:** 250
- **Protein:** 14g
- **Carbohydrates:** 40g
- **Fiber:** 12g
- **Fat:** 2g

Thai-Inspired Vegetable and Tofu Stir-Fry

- **Total Time:** 30 minutes
- **Servings:** 4

Ingredients:

- 1 block extra-firm tofu, pressed and cubed
- 2 cups broccoli florets
- 1 bell pepper, sliced
- 1 carrot, julienned

- 1 zucchini, sliced
- 3 tablespoons soy sauce
- 2 tablespoons peanut butter
- 1 tablespoon maple syrup
- 1 tablespoon sesame oil
- 1 teaspoon ginger, minced
- 2 cloves garlic, minced
- Crushed red pepper flakes (optional)
- Cooked brown rice for serving

Directions:

1. In a wok or skillet, stir-fry tofu until golden. Set aside.
2. Stir-fry broccoli, bell pepper, carrot, and zucchini until tender-crisp.
3. In a bowl, whisk together soy sauce, peanut butter, maple syrup, sesame oil, ginger, garlic, and red pepper flakes.
4. Add tofu and sauce to the vegetables. Toss until coated.
5. Serve over cooked brown rice.

Nutritional Information (per serving):

- **Calories:** 380
- **Protein:** 18g
- **Carbohydrates:** 40g
- **Fiber:** 8g
- **Fat:** 18g

Vegan Stuffed Bell Peppers with Rice and Beans

- **Total Time:** 1 hour
- **Servings:** 4

Ingredients:
- 4 large bell peppers, halved and seeds removed
- 1 cup cooked brown rice
- 1 can black beans, drained and rinsed
- 1 cup corn kernels
- 1 onion, diced
- 1 can diced tomatoes
- 1 teaspoon cumin
- 1 teaspoon chili powder
- Salt and pepper to taste
- Vegan cheese for topping (optional)

Directions:
1. Preheat the oven to 375°F (190°C).
2. In a bowl, mix cooked brown rice, black beans, corn, onion, diced tomatoes, cumin, chili powder, salt, and pepper.
3. Stuff each bell pepper half with the rice and bean mixture.
4. Bake for 30-35 minutes until peppers are tender.
5. Optionally, top with vegan cheese and bake for an additional 5 minutes.

Nutritional Information (per serving):
- **Calories:** 320
- **Protein:** 12g
- **Carbohydrates:** 60g
- **Fiber:** 12g
- **Fat:** 2g

Quinoa and Sweet Potato Stew

- **Total Time:** 40 minutes
- **Servings:** 4

Ingredients:

- 1 cup quinoa, rinsed
- 2 sweet potatoes, peeled and diced
- 1 can chickpeas, drained and rinsed
- 1 onion, chopped
- 3 cloves garlic, minced
- 1 can diced tomatoes
- 4 cups vegetable broth
- 1 teaspoon cumin
- 1 teaspoon smoked paprika
- Salt and pepper to taste
- Fresh cilantro for garnish

Directions:

1. In a pot, sauté onions and garlic until softened.
2. Add quinoa, sweet potatoes, chickpeas, diced tomatoes, vegetable broth, cumin, smoked paprika, salt, and pepper.
3. Bring to a boil, then simmer for 25 minutes.
4. Garnish with fresh cilantro before serving.

Nutritional Information (per serving):

- **Calories:** 380
- **Protein:** 12g
- **Carbohydrates:** 65g
- **Fiber:** 12g
- **Fat:** 6g

Cauliflower and Chickpea Tikka Masala

- **Total Time:** 45 minutes
- **Servings:** 4

Ingredients:

- 1 cauliflower, cut into florets
- 1 can chickpeas, drained and rinsed
- 1 onion, finely chopped
- 3 cloves garlic, minced
- 1 tablespoon ginger, minced
- 1 can diced tomatoes
- 1 can coconut milk
- 2 tablespoons tomato paste
- 2 teaspoons garam masala
- 1 teaspoon turmeric
- 1 teaspoon cumin
- 1/2 teaspoon cayenne pepper (optional)
- Salt and pepper to taste
- Fresh cilantro for garnish
- Cooked basmati rice for serving

Directions:

1. In a pan, sauté onions, garlic, and ginger until softened.
2. Add cauliflower, chickpeas, diced tomatoes, coconut milk, tomato paste, garam masala, turmeric, cumin, cayenne pepper, salt, and pepper.
3. Simmer for 25-30 minutes until the cauliflower is tender.
4. Serve over cooked basmati rice and garnish with fresh cilantro.

Nutritional Information (per serving):
- **Calories:** 420
- **Protein:** 14g
- **Carbohydrates:** 50g
- **Fiber:** 12g
- **Fat:** 20g

Vegan Ratatouille with Quinoa

- **Total Time:** 50 minutes
- **Servings:** 4

Ingredients:
- 1 eggplant, sliced
- 2 zucchinis, sliced
- 1 bell pepper, sliced
- 1 onion, sliced
- 3 cloves garlic, minced
- 1 can diced tomatoes
- 2 tablespoons tomato paste
- 1 teaspoon dried thyme
- 1 teaspoon dried rosemary
- Salt and pepper to taste
- 1 cup quinoa, cooked
- Fresh basil for garnish

Directions:
1. Preheat the oven to 375°F (190°C).
2. In a baking dish, layer sliced eggplant, zucchini, bell pepper, and onion.
3. Mix minced garlic, diced tomatoes, tomato paste, thyme, rosemary, salt, and pepper. Pour over the vegetables.
4. Bake for 30-35 minutes until vegetables are tender.
5. Serve over cooked quinoa and garnish with fresh basil.

Nutritional Information (per serving):
- **Calories:** 320
- **Protein:** 8g
- **Carbohydrates:** 60g
- **Fiber:** 12g
- **Fat:** 4g

Lentil and Mushroom Vegan Shepherd's Pie

- **Total Time:** 1 hour 15 minutes
- **Servings:** 6

Ingredients:
- 2 cups green lentils, cooked
- 1 onion, diced
- 2 carrots, diced
- 2 celery stalks, diced
- 3 cloves garlic, minced
- 8 oz mushrooms, sliced
- 1 cup frozen peas
- 2 tablespoons tomato paste
- 2 tablespoons soy sauce
- 1 teaspoon dried thyme
- 1 teaspoon rosemary
- 4 cups mashed potatoes (prepared separately)
- Olive oil for sautéing
- Salt and pepper to taste

Directions:
1. Preheat the oven to 400°F (200°C).
2. In a skillet, sauté onions, carrots, celery, and garlic until softened.

3. Add mushrooms, lentils, peas, tomato paste, soy sauce, thyme, rosemary, salt, and pepper. Cook for 10 minutes.
4. Transfer the lentil and vegetable mixture to a baking dish.
5. Spread mashed potatoes over the top.
6. Bake for 25-30 minutes until the top is golden brown.

Nutritional Information (per serving):
- **Calories:** 380
- **Protein:** 14g
- **Carbohydrates:** 60g
- **Fiber:** 14g
- **Fat:** 8g

Coconut and Turmeric Lentil Soup

- **Total Time:** 40 minutes
- **Servings:** 4

Ingredients:
- 1 cup red lentils, rinsed
- 1 onion, chopped
- 3 cloves garlic, minced
- 1 teaspoon turmeric
- 1 can coconut milk
- 4 cups vegetable broth
- 1 cup spinach, chopped
- 1 tablespoon coconut oil
- Salt and pepper to taste
- Fresh cilantro for garnish
- Lime wedges for serving

Directions:
1. In a pot, sauté onions and garlic in coconut oil until softened.
2. Add red lentils, turmeric, coconut milk, vegetable broth, salt, and pepper. Simmer for 25-30 minutes.
3. Stir in chopped spinach and cook until wilted.
4. Garnish with fresh cilantro and serve with lime wedges.

Nutritional Information (per serving):
- **Calories:** 320
- **Protein:** 15g
- **Carbohydrates:** 40g
- **Fiber:** 10g
- **Fat:** 14g

Vegetarian and Vegan

Vegan Chickpea Spinach Burgers

- **Total Time:** 30 minutes
- **Servings:** 4

Ingredients:
- 1 can chickpeas, drained and rinsed
- 2 cups fresh spinach, chopped
- 1/2 cup breadcrumbs
- 1/4 cup red onion, finely chopped
- 2 cloves garlic, minced
- 1 teaspoon cumin
- 1 teaspoon paprika
- Salt and pepper to taste
- Olive oil for cooking
- Burger buns and toppings of choice

Directions:
1. In a food processor, combine chickpeas, spinach, breadcrumbs, red onion, garlic, cumin, paprika, salt, and pepper. Pulse until well combined.
2. Form the mixture into burger patties.
3. Heat olive oil in a skillet and cook patties for 3-4 minutes on each side until golden.
4. Serve on burger buns with your favorite toppings.

Nutritional Information (per serving):
- **Calories:** 250
- **Protein:** 10g
- **Carbohydrates:** 40g
- **Fiber:** 8g
- **Fat:** 6g

Eggplant and Tomato Caprese Salad

- **Total Time:** 20 minutes
- **Servings:** 4

Ingredients:
- 1 large eggplant, sliced
- 2 large tomatoes, sliced
- 1 cup vegan mozzarella, sliced
- Fresh basil leaves
- Balsamic glaze
- Olive oil
- Salt and pepper to taste

Directions:
1. Grill or roast eggplant slices until tender.
2. Arrange eggplant, tomato, and mozzarella slices on a serving platter.
3. Tuck fresh basil leaves between the slices.
4. Drizzle with olive oil and balsamic glaze.
5. Sprinkle with salt and pepper before serving.

Nutritional Information (per serving):
- **Calories:** 180
- **Protein:** 8g
- **Carbohydrates:** 15g
- **Fiber:** 6g
- **Fat:** 12g

Vegan Butternut Squash Risotto

- **Total Time:** 45 minutes
- **Servings:** 4

Ingredients:
- 2 cups Arborio rice
- 4 cups vegetable broth, heated
- 1 small butternut squash, diced
- 1 onion, diced
- 2 cloves garlic, minced
- 1/2 cup dry white wine
- 1/2 cup nutritional yeast
- 2 tablespoons olive oil
- Salt and pepper to taste
- Fresh parsley for garnish

Directions:
1. In a pan, sauté onions and garlic in olive oil until softened.
2. Add Arborio rice and cook for 2 minutes.
3. Pour in white wine and stir until absorbed.
4. Gradually add hot vegetable broth, stirring continuously until rice is creamy and cooked.
5. In a separate pan, roast butternut squash until tender.
6. Fold roasted butternut squash and nutritional yeast into the risotto.
7. Season with salt and pepper, garnish with fresh parsley, and serve.

Nutritional Information (per serving):
- **Calories:** 420
- **Protein:** 8g
- **Carbohydrates:** 80g

- **Fiber:** 6g
- **Fat:** 8g

Cauliflower and Chickpea Tacos with Lime Crema

- **Total Time:** 40 minutes
- **Servings:** 4

Ingredients:
- 1 small head cauliflower, cut into florets
- 1 can chickpeas, drained and rinsed
- 1 tablespoon taco seasoning
- 8 small corn tortillas
- 1 cup red cabbage, shredded
- 1 avocado, sliced
- Lime crema: 1/2 cup vegan mayo, 2 tablespoons lime juice, 1 teaspoon agave syrup
- Fresh cilantro for garnish

Directions:
1. Toss cauliflower and chickpeas with taco seasoning.
2. Roast in the oven at 400°F (200°C) for 25 minutes until golden.
3. Warm tortillas and assemble with roasted cauliflower and chickpeas, shredded red cabbage, avocado slices, and lime crema.
4. Garnish with fresh cilantro before serving.

Nutritional Information (per serving):
- **Calories:** 320
- **Protein:** 8g
- **Carbohydrates:** 40g
- **Fiber:** 10g
- **Fat:** 18g

Portobello Mushroom Steaks with Balsamic Glaze

- **Total Time:** 25 minutes
- **Servings:** 2

Ingredients:
- 2 large portobello mushrooms, stems removed
- 3 tablespoons balsamic vinegar
- 2 tablespoons soy sauce
- 2 tablespoons olive oil
- 2 cloves garlic, minced
- 1 teaspoon dried thyme
- Salt and pepper to taste
- Fresh parsley for garnish

Directions:
1. In a bowl, whisk together balsamic vinegar, soy sauce, olive oil, garlic, thyme, salt, and pepper.
2. Marinate portobello mushrooms in the mixture for 10-15 minutes.
3. Grill or pan-sear mushrooms for 5-7 minutes on each side.
4. Drizzle with balsamic glaze from the marinade.
5. Garnish with fresh parsley and serve.

Nutritional Information (per serving):
- **Calories:** 180
- **Protein:** 6g
- **Carbohydrates:** 15g
- **Fiber:** 5g
- **Fat:** 12g

Vegan Spinach and Artichoke Dip

- **Total Time:** 30 minutes
- **Servings:** 6

Ingredients:
- 1 cup raw cashews, soaked in hot water for 1 hour
- 1 cup frozen spinach, thawed and drained
- 1 can artichoke hearts, drained and chopped
- 1/2 cup nutritional yeast
- 1/4 cup vegan mayo
- 2 cloves garlic, minced
- 1 tablespoon lemon juice
- Salt and pepper to taste
- Pita chips or vegetable sticks for dipping

Directions:
1. In a food processor, blend soaked cashews, thawed spinach, chopped artichoke hearts, nutritional yeast, vegan mayo, garlic, lemon juice, salt, and pepper until smooth.
2. Transfer to a serving bowl.
3. Serve with pita chips or vegetable sticks for dipping.

Nutritional Information (per serving):
- **Calories:** 220
- **Protein:** 8g
- **Carbohydrates:** 15g
- **Fiber:** 4g
- **Fat:** 15g

Zucchini and Tomato Gratin

- **Total Time:** 45 minutes
- **Servings:** 4

Ingredients:

- 3 zucchinis, sliced
- 2 tomatoes, sliced
- 1 onion, thinly sliced
- 2 cloves garlic, minced
- 1/2 cup vegan breadcrumbs
- 1/4 cup nutritional yeast
- 2 tablespoons olive oil
- 1 teaspoon dried oregano
- Salt and pepper to taste
- Fresh basil for garnish

Directions:

1. Preheat the oven to 375°F (190°C).
2. In a skillet, sauté onions and garlic in olive oil until softened.
3. In a baking dish, layer sliced zucchini, tomatoes, and sautéed onions and garlic.
4. In a bowl, combine breadcrumbs, nutritional yeast, dried oregano, salt, and pepper. Sprinkle over the vegetables.
5. Bake for 30-35 minutes until the top is golden.
6. Garnish with fresh basil before serving.

Nutritional Information (per serving):

- **Calories:** 180
- **Protein:** 6g
- **Carbohydrates:** 20g
- **Fiber:** 6g
- **Fat:** 10g

Vegan Fajita Bowl with Black Beans and Corn

- **Total Time:** 30 minutes
- **Servings:** 4

Ingredients:
- 2 cups cooked quinoa
- 1 can black beans, drained and rinsed
- 1 cup corn kernels
- 1 bell pepper, sliced
- 1 red onion, sliced
- 1 teaspoon cumin
- 1 teaspoon chili powder
- 1/2 teaspoon smoked paprika
- Salt and pepper to taste
- Guacamole and salsa for serving

Directions:
1. In a skillet, sauté bell pepper and red onion until softened.
2. Add black beans, corn, cumin, chili powder, smoked paprika, salt, and pepper. Cook for 5 minutes.
3. Serve over cooked quinoa and top with guacamole and salsa.

Nutritional Information (per serving):
- **Calories:** 320
- **Protein:** 12g
- **Carbohydrates:** 60g
- **Fiber:** 12g
- **Fat:** 4g

Vegetarian Quinoa Stuffed Bell Peppers

- **Total Time:** 1 hour
- **Servings:** 4

Ingredients:
- 4 bell peppers, halved and seeds removed
- 1 cup cooked quinoa
- 1 can black beans, drained and rinsed
- 1 cup corn kernels
- 1 cup diced tomatoes
- 1 cup shredded vegan cheese
- 1 teaspoon cumin
- 1 teaspoon chili powder
- Salt and pepper to taste
- Fresh cilantro for garnish

Directions:
1. Preheat the oven to 375°F (190°C).
2. In a bowl, mix quinoa, black beans, corn, diced tomatoes, vegan cheese, cumin, chili powder, salt, and pepper.
3. Stuff each bell pepper half with the quinoa mixture.
4. Bake for 30-35 minutes until peppers are tender.
5. Garnish with fresh cilantro before serving.

Nutritional Information (per serving):
- **Calories:** 280
- **Protein:** 10g
- **Carbohydrates:** 45g
- **Fiber:** 10g
- **Fat:** 8g

Sweet Potato and Black Bean Enchiladas

- **Total Time:** 45 minutes
- **Servings:** 4

Ingredients:
- 2 large sweet potatoes, peeled and diced
- 1 can black beans, drained and rinsed
- 1 cup corn kernels
- 1 red onion, diced
- 2 teaspoons cumin
- 1 teaspoon chili powder
- 1/2 teaspoon smoked paprika
- 8 whole wheat or corn tortillas
- 1 can enchilada sauce
- 1 cup vegan cheese, shredded
- Fresh cilantro for garnish

Directions:
1. Steam or boil sweet potatoes until tender.
2. In a bowl, mash sweet potatoes and mix with black beans, corn, red onion, cumin, chili powder, and smoked paprika.
3. Spoon the mixture onto each tortilla, roll, and place in a baking dish.
4. Pour enchilada sauce over the rolled tortillas and sprinkle with vegan cheese.
5. Bake for 20-25 minutes until bubbly.
6. Garnish with fresh cilantro before serving.

Nutritional Information (per serving):
- **Calories:** 380
- **Protein:** 12g

- **Carbohydrates:** 60g
- **Fiber:** 12g
- **Fat:** 8g

Vegan Lentil and Mushroom Meatballs

- **Total Time:** 40 minutes
- **Servings:** 4

Ingredients:
- 1 cup cooked green lentils
- 8 oz mushrooms, finely chopped
- 1 onion, finely chopped
- 2 cloves garlic, minced
- 1 cup breadcrumbs
- 1/4 cup nutritional yeast
- 1 tablespoon soy sauce
- 1 teaspoon dried oregano
- 1 teaspoon dried basil
- Olive oil for baking
- Marinara sauce for serving

Directions:
1. Preheat the oven to 375°F (190°C).
2. In a pan, sauté mushrooms, onions, and garlic until softened.
3. In a bowl, mix cooked lentils, sautéed mushrooms and onions, breadcrumbs, nutritional yeast, soy sauce, oregano, and basil.
4. Form the mixture into meatballs and place on a baking sheet.
5. Bake for 20-25 minutes until golden.
6. Serve with marinara sauce.

Nutritional Information (per serving):
- **Calories:** 320
- **Protein:** 14g
- **Carbohydrates:** 45g
- **Fiber:** 10g
- **Fat:** 6g

Vegan Eggplant Parmesan

- **Total Time:** 1 hour
- **Servings:** 4

Ingredients:
- 1 large eggplant, sliced
- 1 cup whole wheat breadcrumbs
- 1/2 cup nutritional yeast
- 1 teaspoon dried oregano
- 1 teaspoon dried basil
- 2 cups marinara sauce
- 1 cup vegan mozzarella, shredded
- Fresh basil for garnish

Directions:
1. Preheat the oven to 375°F (190°C).
2. In a bowl, mix breadcrumbs, nutritional yeast, oregano, and basil.
3. Dredge each eggplant slice in the breadcrumb mixture and place on a baking sheet.
4. Bake for 25-30 minutes until the eggplant is tender.
5. In a baking dish, layer marinara sauce, baked eggplant slices, and vegan mozzarella.
6. Repeat the layers and bake for an additional 20 minutes until bubbly.
7. Garnish with fresh basil before serving.

Nutritional Information (per serving):

- **Calories:** 280
- **Protein:** 10g
- **Carbohydrates:** 45g
- **Fiber:** 12g
- **Fat:** 6g

Mediterranean Chickpea Wrap

- **Total Time:** 15 minutes
- **Servings:** 2

Ingredients:

- 1 can chickpeas, drained and rinsed
- 1/2 cup cherry tomatoes, halved
- 1/4 cup red onion, finely chopped
- 1/4 cup cucumber, diced
- 1/4 cup Kalamata olives, sliced
- 1/4 cup fresh parsley, chopped
- 2 whole wheat wraps
- 2 tablespoons hummus
- Lemon-tahini dressing (1/4 cup tahini, 2 tablespoons lemon juice, 1 clove garlic, minced, salt, and pepper)

Directions:

1. In a bowl, mix chickpeas, cherry tomatoes, red onion, cucumber, olives, and parsley.
2. Warm the wraps and spread each with hummus.
3. Spoon the chickpea mixture onto the wraps and drizzle with lemon-tahini dressing.
4. Fold the wraps and serve.

Nutritional Information (per serving):
- **Calories:** 320
- **Protein:** 10g
- **Carbohydrates:** 50g
- **Fiber:** 12g
- **Fat:** 10g

Stuffed Portobello Mushrooms with Quinoa and Pesto

- **Total Time:** 40 minutes
- **Servings:** 4

Ingredients:
- 4 large portobello mushrooms, stems removed
- 1 cup cooked quinoa
- 1 cup cherry tomatoes, halved
- 1/2 cup vegan pesto
- 1/4 cup pine nuts, toasted
- Fresh basil for garnish

Directions:
1. Preheat the oven to 375°F (190°C).
2. Place portobello mushrooms on a baking sheet.
3. In a bowl, mix cooked quinoa, cherry tomatoes, and half of the vegan pesto.
4. Stuff each mushroom with the quinoa mixture.
5. Drizzle the remaining pesto over the mushrooms and bake for 25-30 minutes.
6. Garnish with toasted pine nuts and fresh basil before serving.

Nutritional Information (per serving):
- **Calories:** 320

- **Protein:** 12g
- **Carbohydrates:** 40g
- **Fiber:** 8g
- **Fat:** 14g

Vegan Greek Salad with Tofu Feta

- **Total Time:** 20 minutes
- **Servings:** 4

Ingredients:
- 1 block firm tofu, pressed and cubed
- 2 tablespoons olive oil
- 1 tablespoon lemon juice
- 1 teaspoon dried oregano
- Salt and pepper to taste
- 2 cups cherry tomatoes, halved
- 1 cucumber, diced
- 1 red onion, thinly sliced
- 1 cup Kalamata olives, sliced
- 1/2 cup vegan Greek dressing (2 tablespoons olive oil, 1 tablespoon red wine vinegar, 1 teaspoon Dijon mustard, 1 teaspoon maple syrup, 1 clove garlic, minced)

Directions:
1. In a bowl, toss cubed tofu with olive oil, lemon juice, oregano, salt, and pepper. Allow to marinate for at least 10 minutes.
2. In a large salad bowl, combine cherry tomatoes, cucumber, red onion, and Kalamata olives.
3. Add marinated tofu to the salad.

4. In a small bowl, whisk together olive oil, red wine vinegar, Dijon mustard, maple syrup, and minced garlic to create the dressing.
5. Drizzle the dressing over the salad and toss gently before serving.

Nutritional Information (per serving):
- **Calories:** 280
- **Protein:** 12g
- **Carbohydrates:** 25g
- **Fiber:** 8g
- **Fat:** 18g

Snacks and Sides

Baked Sweet Potato Fries with Garlic Aioli

- **Total Time:** 40 minutes
- **Servings:** 4

Ingredients:
- 2 large sweet potatoes, cut into fries
- 2 tablespoons olive oil
- 1 teaspoon smoked paprika
- 1/2 teaspoon garlic powder
- Salt and pepper to taste

Garlic Aioli:
- 1/2 cup vegan mayo
- 2 cloves garlic, minced
- 1 tablespoon lemon juice
- Salt and pepper to taste

Directions:
1. Preheat the oven to 425°F (220°C).
2. In a bowl, toss sweet potato fries with olive oil, smoked paprika, garlic powder, salt, and pepper.
3. Spread the fries in a single layer on a baking sheet and bake for 30-35 minutes until crispy.
4. For the garlic aioli, whisk together vegan mayo, minced garlic, lemon juice, salt, and pepper.
5. Serve the sweet potato fries with the garlic aioli for dipping.

Nutritional Information (per serving):
- **Calories:** 220

- **Protein:** 2g
- **Carbohydrates:** 30g
- **Fiber:** 5g
- **Fat:** 10g

Vegan Guacamole with Whole Grain Chips

- **Total Time:** 15 minutes
- **Servings:** 6

Ingredients:
- 3 ripe avocados, mashed
- 1 tomato, diced
- 1/4 cup red onion, finely chopped
- 1/4 cup fresh cilantro, chopped
- 1 lime, juiced
- Salt and pepper to taste
- Whole grain tortilla chips for serving

Directions:
1. In a bowl, combine mashed avocados, diced tomato, chopped red onion, cilantro, lime juice, salt, and pepper.
2. Mix until well combined.
3. Serve with whole grain tortilla chips.

Nutritional Information (per serving):
- **Calories:** 180
- **Protein:** 3g
- **Carbohydrates:** 15g
- **Fiber:** 8g
- **Fat:** 14g

Roasted Chickpeas with Smoky Paprika

- **Total Time:** 30 minutes
- **Servings:** 4

Ingredients:
- 2 cans chickpeas, drained and rinsed
- 2 tablespoons olive oil
- 1 teaspoon smoked paprika
- 1/2 teaspoon cayenne pepper
- Salt to taste

Directions:
1. Preheat the oven to 400°F (200°C).
2. Pat chickpeas dry with a paper towel and toss with olive oil, smoked paprika, cayenne pepper, and salt.
3. Spread chickpeas on a baking sheet and roast for 20-25 minutes until crispy.
4. Allow to cool before serving.

Nutritional Information (per serving):
- **Calories:** 220
- **Protein:** 9g
- **Carbohydrates:** 30g
- **Fiber:** 8g
- **Fat:** 8g

Spicy Edamame with Sea Salt

- **Total Time:** 10 minutes
- **Servings:** 4

Ingredients:
- 2 cups edamame, steamed
- 1 tablespoon sesame oil
- 1 teaspoon soy sauce
- 1/2 teaspoon chili flakes
- Sea salt to taste

Directions:
1. In a bowl, toss steamed edamame with sesame oil, soy sauce, chili flakes, and sea salt.
2. Serve warm.

Nutritional Information (per serving):
- **Calories:** 160
- **Protein:** 12g
- **Carbohydrates:** 10g
- **Fiber:** 5g
- **Fat:** 10g

Vegan Spinach and Artichoke Stuffed Mushrooms

- **Total Time:** 25 minutes
- **Servings:** 6

Ingredients:
- 12 large mushrooms, stems removed
- 1 cup fresh spinach, chopped
- 1 can artichoke hearts, drained and chopped

- 1/2 cup vegan cream cheese
- 1/4 cup nutritional yeast
- 2 cloves garlic, minced
- Salt and pepper to taste
- Fresh parsley for garnish

Directions:
1. Preheat the oven to 375°F (190°C).
2. In a bowl, mix chopped spinach, chopped artichoke hearts, vegan cream cheese, nutritional yeast, minced garlic, salt, and pepper.
3. Stuff each mushroom cap with the spinach and artichoke mixture.
4. Bake for 15-20 minutes until mushrooms are tender.
5. Garnish with fresh parsley before serving.

Nutritional Information (per serving):
- **Calories:** 120
- **Protein:** 6g
- **Carbohydrates:** 10g
- **Fiber:** 3g
- **Fat:** 8g

Turmeric Hummus with Crudites

- **Total Time:** 15 minutes
- **Servings:** 8

Ingredients:
- 2 cans chickpeas, drained and rinsed
- 1/4 cup tahini
- 1/4 cup olive oil
- 2 cloves garlic, minced

- 1 teaspoon ground turmeric
- 1 teaspoon cumin
- Juice of 1 lemon
- Salt and pepper to taste
- Assorted crudites (carrot sticks, cucumber slices, cherry tomatoes) for dipping

Directions:
1. In a food processor, blend chickpeas, tahini, olive oil, minced garlic, ground turmeric, cumin, lemon juice, salt, and pepper until smooth.
2. Adjust seasoning to taste.
3. Serve with assorted crudites for dipping.

Nutritional Information (per serving):
- **Calories:** 180
- **Protein:** 6g
- **Carbohydrates:** 15g
- **Fiber:** 5g
- **Fat:** 10g

Vegan Pesto Zucchini Noodles

- **Total Time:** 20 minutes
- **Servings:** 4

Ingredients:
- 4 medium zucchinis, spiralized
- 1 cup cherry tomatoes, halved
- 1/2 cup vegan pesto
- 1/4 cup pine nuts, toasted
- Fresh basil for garnish
- Salt and pepper to taste

Directions:
1. In a pan, sauté spiralized zucchini until just tender.
2. Toss zucchini noodles with cherry tomatoes, vegan pesto, toasted pine nuts, salt, and pepper.
3. Garnish with fresh basil before serving.

Nutritional Information (per serving):
- **Calories:** 150
- **Protein:** 5g
- **Carbohydrates:** 10g
- **Fiber:** 3g
- **Fat:** 10g

Avocado and Black Bean Salsa

- **Total Time:** 15 minutes
- **Servings:** 6

Ingredients:
- 2 avocados, diced
- 1 can black beans, drained and rinsed
- 1 cup corn kernels
- 1/4 cup red onion, finely chopped
- 1/4 cup fresh cilantro, chopped
- Juice of 2 limes
- Salt and pepper to taste

Directions:
1. In a bowl, combine diced avocados, black beans, corn, chopped red onion, cilantro, lime juice, salt, and pepper.
2. Mix gently until well combined.
3. Serve as a salsa with tortilla chips or as a side dish.

Nutritional Information (per serving):
- **Calories:** 180
- **Protein:** 6g
- **Carbohydrates:** 25g
- **Fiber:** 8g
- **Fat:** 8g

Vegan Buffalo Cauliflower Bites

- **Total Time:** 35 minutes
- **Servings:** 4

Ingredients:
- 1 head cauliflower, cut into florets
- 1 cup almond flour
- 1 cup plant-based milk
- 1 teaspoon garlic powder
- 1 teaspoon onion powder
- 1/2 cup buffalo sauce
- Vegan ranch dressing for dipping

Directions:
1. Preheat the oven to 450°F (230°C).
2. In a bowl, mix almond flour, plant-based milk, garlic powder, and onion powder to create a batter.
3. Dip cauliflower florets into the batter and place them on a baking sheet.
4. Bake for 20 minutes until golden.
5. Toss baked cauliflower in buffalo sauce.
6. Serve with vegan ranch dressing for dipping.

Nutritional Information (per serving):
- **Calories:** 220
- **Protein:** 8g

- **Carbohydrates:** 20g
- **Fiber:** 6g
- **Fat:** 12g

Cucumber and Tomato Salad with Dill Dressing

- **Total Time:** 15 minutes
- **Servings:** 4

Ingredients:
- 2 cucumbers, thinly sliced
- 2 cups cherry tomatoes, halved
- 1/4 cup red onion, thinly sliced
- 1/4 cup fresh dill, chopped
- 2 tablespoons olive oil
- 1 tablespoon red wine vinegar
- Salt and pepper to taste

Directions:
1. In a bowl, combine sliced cucumbers, halved cherry tomatoes, sliced red onion, and chopped fresh dill.
2. In a small bowl, whisk together olive oil, red wine vinegar, salt, and pepper to create the dressing.
3. Pour the dressing over the salad and toss gently before serving.

Nutritional Information (per serving):
- **Calories:** 120
- **Protein:** 2g
- **Carbohydrates:** 10g
- **Fiber:** 3g
- **Fat:** 8g

Dessert

Vegan Chocolate Avocado Mousse

- **Total Time:** 15 minutes
- **Servings:** 4

Ingredients:
- 2 ripe avocados
- 1/4 cup cocoa powder
- 1/4 cup maple syrup
- 1 teaspoon vanilla extract
- A pinch of salt
- Fresh berries for garnish

Directions:
1. In a blender, combine avocados, cocoa powder, maple syrup, vanilla extract, and a pinch of salt.
2. Blend until smooth and creamy.
3. Divide the mousse into serving bowls and refrigerate for at least 1 hour.
4. Garnish with fresh berries before serving.

Nutritional Information (per serving):
- **Calories:** 150
- **Protein:** 2g
- **Carbohydrates:** 20g
- **Fiber:** 6g
- **Fat:** 8g

Berry and Almond Butter Stuffed Dates

- **Total Time:** 10 minutes
- **Servings:** 8

Ingredients:
- 16 Medjool dates, pitted
- 1/4 cup almond butter
- 1/2 cup mixed berries (blueberries, raspberries, or strawberries)

Directions:
1. Gently open each date and remove the pit.
2. Fill each date with a teaspoon of almond butter.
3. Top with mixed berries.
4. Serve immediately or refrigerate until ready to enjoy.

Nutritional Information (per serving):
- **Calories:** 120
- **Protein:** 2g
- **Carbohydrates:** 25g
- **Fiber:** 4g
- **Fat:** 4g

Turmeric Coconut Bliss Balls

- **Total Time:** 20 minutes
- **Servings:** 12

Ingredients:
- 1 cup shredded coconut
- 1/2 cup almond flour

- 1/4 cup maple syrup
- 1 teaspoon turmeric powder
- 1/2 teaspoon vanilla extract
- A pinch of black pepper
- Coconut flakes for rolling

Directions:
1. In a food processor, combine shredded coconut, almond flour, maple syrup, turmeric powder, vanilla extract, and black pepper.
2. Process until the mixture sticks together.
3. Roll the mixture into small balls and coat with coconut flakes.
4. Refrigerate for at least 30 minutes before serving.

Nutritional Information (per serving):
- **Calories:** 80
- **Protein:** 1g
- **Carbohydrates:** 8g
- **Fiber:** 2g
- **Fat:** 5g

Vegan Banana Ice Cream with Pistachios

- **Total Time:** 5 minutes
- **Servings:** 2

Ingredients:
- 3 ripe bananas, sliced and frozen
- 1/4 cup plant-based milk
- 1/4 cup chopped pistachios

Directions:
1. In a blender, combine frozen banana slices and plant-based milk.
2. Blend until smooth and creamy.
3. Scoop the banana ice cream into bowls and top with chopped pistachios.
4. Serve immediately.

Nutritional Information (per serving):
- **Calories:** 180
- **Protein:** 3g
- **Carbohydrates:** 30g
- **Fiber:** 4g
- **Fat:** 7g

Chocolate Chia Seed Pudding

- **Total Time:** 4 hours (including chilling time)
- **Servings:** 4

Ingredients:
- 1/2 cup chia seeds
- 2 cups plant-based milk
- 1/4 cup cocoa powder
- 3 tablespoons maple syrup
- 1 teaspoon vanilla extract
- Vegan chocolate chips for garnish (optional)

Directions:
1. In a bowl, whisk together chia seeds, plant-based milk, cocoa powder, maple syrup, and vanilla extract.
2. Let the mixture sit for 5 minutes, then whisk again to avoid clumps.

3. Cover and refrigerate for at least 4 hours or overnight.
4. Stir before serving and garnish with vegan chocolate chips if desired.

Nutritional Information (per serving):
- **Calories:** 180
- **Protein:** 5g
- **Carbohydrates:** 20g
- **Fiber:** 8g
- **Fat:** 9g

Vegan Lemon Blueberry Cheesecake Bars

- **Total Time:** 1 hour (including chilling time)
- **Servings:** 9

Ingredients:
- 1 cup raw cashews, soaked for 4 hours
- 1/2 cup coconut cream
- 1/4 cup lemon juice
- 1/4 cup maple syrup
- 1 teaspoon vanilla extract
- 1 cup fresh blueberries
- 1 cup almond flour
- 1/4 cup coconut oil, melted
- 2 tablespoons maple syrup

Directions:
1. Preheat the oven to 350°F (175°C) and line a square baking dish with parchment paper.

2. In a food processor, combine soaked cashews, coconut cream, lemon juice, maple syrup, and vanilla extract. Blend until smooth.

3. In a bowl, mix almond flour, melted coconut oil, and maple syrup. Press the mixture into the bottom of the prepared baking dish.

4. Spread the cashew mixture over the crust and top with fresh blueberries.

5. Refrigerate for at least 3 hours before slicing into bars.

Nutritional Information (per serving):
- **Calories:** 280
- **Protein:** 6g
- **Carbohydrates:** 20g
- **Fiber:** 3g
- **Fat:** 21g

Almond Flour and Berry Crisp

- **Total Time:** 45 minutes
- **Servings:** 6

Ingredients:
- 3 cups mixed berries (strawberries, blueberries, raspberries)
- 2 tablespoons maple syrup
- 1 teaspoon vanilla extract
- 1 cup almond flour
- 1/4 cup coconut oil, melted
- 1/4 cup maple syrup
- 1/4 cup sliced almonds

Directions:

1. Preheat the oven to 350°F (175°C).
2. In a bowl, toss mixed berries with maple syrup and vanilla extract. Transfer to a baking dish.
3. In a separate bowl, combine almond flour, melted coconut oil, maple syrup, and sliced almonds. Mix until crumbly.
4. Sprinkle the almond flour mixture over the berries.
5. Bake for 30-35 minutes until the topping is golden brown.
6. Allow to cool slightly before serving.

Nutritional Information (per serving):

- **Calories:** 240
- **Protein:** 4g
- **Carbohydrates:** 25g
- **Fiber:** 6g
- **Fat:** 15g

Coconut and Mango Sorbet

- **Total Time:** 5 hours (including freezing time)
- **Servings:** 4

Ingredients:

- 2 cups frozen mango chunks
- 1 can coconut milk
- 1/4 cup agave syrup
- Shredded coconut for garnish

Directions:

1. In a blender, combine frozen mango chunks, coconut milk, and agave syrup.
2. Blend until smooth.

3. Pour the mixture into a shallow dish and freeze for at least 4 hours.
4. Before serving, let the sorbet sit at room temperature for a few minutes, then scoop into bowls.
5. Garnish with shredded coconut.

Nutritional Information (per serving):
- **Calories:** 220
- **Protein:** 2g
- **Carbohydrates:** 30g
- **Fiber:** 3g
- **Fat:** 11g

Vegan Pumpkin Pie with Oat Crust

- **Total Time:** 1 hour 30 minutes
- **Servings:** 8

Ingredients:
Oat Crust:
- 1 1/2 cups rolled oats
- 1/2 cup almond flour
- 1/4 cup coconut oil, melted
- 1/4 cup maple syrup
- A pinch of salt

Pumpkin Filling:
- 1 can pumpkin puree
- 1/2 cup coconut milk
- 1/2 cup maple syrup
- 1 teaspoon vanilla extract
- 1 teaspoon pumpkin pie spice
- A pinch of salt

Directions:

Oat Crust:

1. Preheat the oven to 350°F (175°C) and grease a pie dish.
2. In a food processor, blend rolled oats until they resemble flour.
3. In a bowl, combine oat flour, almond flour, melted coconut oil, maple syrup, and a pinch of salt.
4. Press the mixture into the pie dish, forming a crust.
5. Bake for 10-12 minutes until golden brown.

Pumpkin Filling:

1. In a bowl, whisk together pumpkin puree, coconut milk, maple syrup, vanilla extract, pumpkin pie spice, and a pinch of salt.
2. Pour the pumpkin filling into the baked oat crust.
3. Bake for 50-60 minutes until the filling is set.
4. Allow to cool before slicing and serving.

Nutritional Information (per serving):

- **Calories:** 280
- **Protein:** 5g
- **Carbohydrates:** 30g
- **Fiber:** 4g
- **Fat:** 16g

Avocado Chocolate Mousse Tart

- **Total Time:** 1 hour 30 minutes
- **Servings:** 8

Ingredients:

Chocolate Crust:

- 1 1/2 cups almond flour
- 1/4 cup cocoa powder

- 1/4 cup coconut oil, melted
- 2 tablespoons maple syrup
- A pinch of salt

Avocado Chocolate Mousse:

- 2 ripe avocados
- 1/2 cup cocoa powder
- 1/2 cup maple syrup
- 1 teaspoon vanilla extract
- A pinch of salt

Directions:

Chocolate Crust:

1. Preheat the oven to 350°F (175°C) and grease a tart pan.
2. In a bowl, mix almond flour, cocoa powder, melted coconut oil, maple syrup, and a pinch of salt.
3. Press the mixture into the tart pan to form a crust.
4. Bake for 12-15 minutes until the crust is set.

Avocado Chocolate Mousse:

1. In a blender, combine ripe avocados, cocoa powder, maple syrup, vanilla extract, and a pinch of salt.
2. Blend until smooth and creamy.
3. Once the crust is cooled, spread the avocado chocolate mousse over it.
4. Refrigerate for at least 1 hour before slicing and serving.

Nutritional Information (per serving):

- **Calories:** 260
- **Protein:** 4g
- **Carbohydrates:** 30g
- **Fiber:** 6g
- **Fat:** 16g

Smoothie

Green Detox Smoothie with Kale and Pineapple

- **Total Time:** 5 minutes
- **Servings:** 2

Ingredients:
- 2 cups kale, stems removed
- 1 cup pineapple chunks
- 1 green apple, cored and chopped
- 1 cucumber, peeled and sliced
- 1 tablespoon chia seeds
- 1 cup coconut water
- Ice cubes (optional)

Directions:
1. In a blender, combine kale, pineapple chunks, green apple, cucumber, chia seeds, and coconut water.
2. Blend until smooth.
3. Add ice cubes if desired and blend again.
4. Pour into glasses and enjoy.

Nutritional Information (per serving):
- **Calories:** 120
- **Protein:** 3g
- **Carbohydrates:** 25g
- **Fiber:** 7g
- **Fat:** 2g

Berry Blast Smoothie with Almond Milk

- **Total Time:** 5 minutes
- **Servings:** 2

Ingredients:
- 1 cup mixed berries (strawberries, blueberries, raspberries)
- 1 banana, peeled
- 1 cup almond milk
- 1 tablespoon hemp seeds
- 1 teaspoon agave syrup
- Ice cubes (optional)

Directions:
1. In a blender, combine mixed berries, banana, almond milk, hemp seeds, and agave syrup.
2. Blend until smooth.
3. Add ice cubes if desired and blend again.
4. Pour into glasses and enjoy.

Nutritional Information (per serving):
- **Calories:** 150
- **Protein:** 4g
- **Carbohydrates:** 30g
- **Fiber:** 6g
- **Fat:** 3g

Mango Turmeric Smoothie

- **Total Time:** 5 minutes
- **Servings:** 2

Ingredients:
- 2 cups fresh or frozen mango chunks
- 1 banana, peeled
- 1 teaspoon turmeric powder
- 1/2 teaspoon ginger, grated
- 1 cup coconut water
- 1 tablespoon chia seeds
- Ice cubes (optional)

Directions:
1. In a blender, combine mango chunks, banana, turmeric powder, grated ginger, coconut water, and chia seeds.
2. Blend until smooth.
3. Add ice cubes if desired and blend again.
4. Pour into glasses and enjoy.

Nutritional Information (per serving):
- **Calories:** 180
- **Protein:** 3g
- **Carbohydrates:** 35g
- **Fiber:** 6g
- **Fat:** 2g

Blueberry Spinach Protein Smoothie

- **Total Time:** 5 minutes
- **Servings:** 2

Ingredients:
- 1 cup blueberries, fresh or frozen
- 2 cups baby spinach
- 1 scoop plant-based protein powder
- 1 tablespoon almond butter
- 1 cup almond milk
- 1 tablespoon flaxseeds
- Ice cubes (optional)

Directions:
1. In a blender, combine blueberries, baby spinach, plant-based protein powder, almond butter, almond milk, and flaxseeds.
2. Blend until smooth.
3. Add ice cubes if desired and blend again.
4. Pour into glasses and enjoy.

Nutritional Information (per serving):
- **Calories:** 250
- **Protein:** 15g
- **Carbohydrates:** 25g
- **Fiber:** 8g
- **Fat:** 10g

Pineapple and Ginger Energizing Smoothie

- **Total Time:** 5 minutes
- **Servings:** 2

Ingredients:
- 2 cups pineapple chunks
- 1 inch ginger, peeled and grated
- 1 banana, peeled
- 1 cup coconut water
- 1 tablespoon chia seeds
- 1 teaspoon honey or agave syrup
- Ice cubes (optional)

Directions:
1. In a blender, combine pineapple chunks, grated ginger, banana, coconut water, chia seeds, and honey or agave syrup.
2. Blend until smooth.
3. Add ice cubes if desired and blend again.
4. Pour into glasses and enjoy.

Nutritional Information (per serving):
- **Calories:** 160
- **Protein:** 3g
- **Carbohydrates:** 35g
- **Fiber:** 7g
- **Fat:** 2g

Vegan Chocolate Protein Smoothie

- **Total Time:** 5 minutes
- **Servings:** 2

Ingredients:
- 2 cups plant-based chocolate protein milk
- 1 banana, peeled
- 2 tablespoons almond butter
- 1 tablespoon chia seeds
- 1 teaspoon cacao powder
- Ice cubes (optional)

Directions:
1. In a blender, combine plant-based chocolate protein milk, banana, almond butter, chia seeds, and cacao powder.
2. Blend until smooth.
3. Add ice cubes if desired and blend again.
4. Pour into glasses and enjoy.

Nutritional Information (per serving):
- **Calories:** 280
- **Protein:** 15g
- **Carbohydrates:** 30g
- **Fiber:** 8g
- **Fat:** 12g

Peach and Turmeric Anti-Inflammatory Smoothie

- **Total Time:** 5 minutes
- **Servings:** 2

Ingredients:

- 2 cups fresh or frozen peaches
- 1 teaspoon turmeric powder
- 1/2 teaspoon cinnamon
- 1 cup almond milk
- 1 tablespoon hemp seeds
- 1 teaspoon honey or agave syrup
- Ice cubes (optional)

Directions:

1. In a blender, combine peaches, turmeric powder, cinnamon, almond milk, hemp seeds, and honey or agave syrup.
2. Blend until smooth.
3. Add ice cubes if desired and blend again.
4. Pour into glasses and enjoy.

Nutritional Information (per serving):

- **Calories:** 150
- **Protein:** 4g
- **Carbohydrates:** 30g
- **Fiber:** 6g
- **Fat:** 3g

Avocado Mint Green Smoothie

- **Total Time:** 5 minutes
- **Servings:** 2

Ingredients:
- 1 ripe avocado, peeled and pitted
- 1 cup spinach leaves
- 1/2 cup fresh mint leaves
- 1 banana, peeled
- 1 cup coconut water
- 1 tablespoon chia seeds
- Ice cubes (optional)

Directions:
1. In a blender, combine ripe avocado, spinach leaves, fresh mint leaves, banana, coconut water, and chia seeds.
2. Blend until smooth.
3. Add ice cubes if desired and blend again.
4. Pour into glasses and enjoy.

Nutritional Information (per serving):
- **Calories:** 200
- **Protein:** 4g
- **Carbohydrates:** 30g
- **Fiber:** 9g
- **Fat:** 8g

Golden Mango Lassi with Turmeric

- **Total Time:** 5 minutes
- **Servings:** 2

Ingredients:

- 2 cups fresh or frozen mango chunks
- 1 cup plain coconut yogurt
- 1 teaspoon turmeric powder
- 1/2 teaspoon cardamom
- 1 tablespoon maple syrup
- 1/2 cup water
- Ice cubes (optional)

Directions:

1. In a blender, combine mango chunks, coconut yogurt, turmeric powder, cardamom, maple syrup, and water.
2. Blend until smooth.
3. Add ice cubes if desired and blend again.
4. Pour into glasses and enjoy.

Nutritional Information (per serving):

- **Calories:** 180
- **Protein:** 2g
- **Carbohydrates:** 35g
- **Fiber:** 5g
- **Fat:** 3g

Raspberry and Almond Butter Protein Smoothie

- **Total Time:** 5 minutes
- **Servings:** 2

Ingredients:
- 1 cup raspberries, fresh or frozen
- 2 tablespoons almond butter
- 1 scoop plant-based protein powder
- 1 banana, peeled
- 1 cup almond milk
- 1 tablespoon flaxseeds
- Ice cubes (optional)

Directions:
1. In a blender, combine raspberries, almond butter, plant-based protein powder, banana, almond milk, and flaxseeds.
2. Blend until smooth.
3. Add ice cubes if desired and blend again.
4. Pour into glasses and enjoy.

Nutritional Information (per serving):
- **Calories:** 260
- **Protein:** 15g
- **Carbohydrates:** 25g
- **Fiber:** 8g
- **Fat:** 10g

14-Day Meal Plan

Day 1:
- **Breakfast:** Vegan Pancakes with Maple Syrup and Pecans
- **Lunch:** Sweet Potato and Kale Salad with Avocado
- **Dinner:** Eggplant and Lentil Moussaka

Day 2:
- **Breakfast:** Mango Turmeric Smoothie
- **Lunch:** Vegan BBQ Jackfruit Tacos
- **Dinner:** Vegan Mushroom and Spinach Lasagna

Day 3:
- **Breakfast:** Almond Butter and Banana Breakfast Wrap
- **Lunch:** Broccoli and Quinoa Patties
- **Dinner:** Spaghetti Squash Primavera with Vegan Pesto

Day 4:
- **Breakfast:** Vegan French Toast with Cinnamon and Maple Syrup
- **Lunch:** Vegan Chickpea and Vegetable Stir-Fry
- **Dinner:** Chickpea and Vegetable Coconut Curry

Day 5:
- **Breakfast:** Green Tea Infused Overnight Oats
- **Lunch:** Brown Rice and Black Bean Burrito Bowl
- **Dinner:** Stuffed Acorn Squash with Quinoa and Cranberries

Day 6:
- **Breakfast:** Berry and Spinach Smoothie
- **Lunch:** Zucchini Noodles with Pesto and Cherry Tomatoes
- **Dinner:** Roasted Brussels Sprouts and Cauliflower Tacos

Day 7:
- **Breakfast:** Vegan Chocolate Protein Smoothie
- **Lunch:** Sweet Potato and Chickpea Buddha Bowl
- **Dinner:** Cabbage and Lentil Soup

Day 8:
- **Breakfast:** Vegan Pancakes with Maple Syrup and Pecans
- **Lunch:** Quinoa and Black Bean Stuffed Peppers
- **Dinner:** Vegan Lentil Loaf with Tomato Glaze

Day 9:
- **Breakfast:** Mango Turmeric Smoothie
- **Lunch:** Vegan Chickpea and Vegetable Stir-Fry
- **Dinner:** Vegan Ratatouille with Quinoa

Day 10:
- **Breakfast:** Vegan French Toast with Cinnamon and Maple Syrup
- **Lunch:** Brown Rice and Black Bean Burrito Bowl
- **Dinner:** Coconut and Turmeric Lentil Soup

Day 11:
- **Breakfast:** Green Tea Infused Overnight Oats
- **Lunch:** Broccoli and Quinoa Patties
- **Dinner:** Quinoa and Sweet Potato Stew

Day 12:
- **Breakfast:** Berry and Spinach Smoothie
- **Lunch:** Mediterranean Chickpea Salad
- **Dinner:** Vegan Mushroom and Spinach Lasagna

Day 13:
- **Breakfast:** Avocado Toast with Cherry Tomatoes and Microgreens
- **Lunch:** Vegan BBQ Jackfruit Tacos
- **Dinner:** Eggplant and Lentil Moussaka

Day 14:
- **Breakfast:** Vegan Chocolate Protein Smoothie
- **Lunch:** Zucchini Noodles with Pesto and Cherry Tomatoes
- **Dinner:** Stuffed Acorn Squash with Quinoa and Cranberries

Conclusion

As you reach the conclusion of this plant-based anti-inflammatory cookbook, it's essential to recognize that what you have embarked upon is not just a temporary shift in your diet but a profound transformation—a commitment to a lifelong journey towards health and well-being. This journey is not merely about the food you consume; it encompasses a holistic approach to nourishing your body, mind, and spirit.

Take a moment to reflect on the remarkable journey you've undertaken. You've explored a diverse array of plant-based recipes, each meticulously crafted to not only tantalize your taste buds but to also harness the power of natural, anti-inflammatory ingredients. Your commitment to choosing plant-based options has not only contributed to your personal health but has also played a role in the larger narrative of sustainable living and environmental consciousness.

Consider the positive changes you may have noticed—increased energy levels, improved digestion, and perhaps a newfound sense of vitality. Your body has been receiving a rich influx of nutrients, antioxidants, and wholesome goodness from the plant-based ingredients, and it's responding with resilience and vitality.

Celebrating your successes, no matter how small, is an integral part of this journey. Whether you've mastered a particular recipe, successfully navigated social situations while adhering to your plant-based lifestyle, or simply noticed positive changes in your well-being, each achievement is a testament to your dedication.

It's equally crucial to acknowledge the challenges you may have encountered. Perhaps there were moments of temptation, social pressures, or instances where finding plant-based options seemed challenging. These moments are not setbacks but opportunities for growth and learning. Reflect on them with kindness and curiosity, understanding that the journey to health is dynamic, and adapting to challenges is an inherent part of the process.

As you conclude this cookbook, remember that this is not the end but a continuation of your journey towards sustained well-being. Continue to explore new recipes, experiment with flavors, and discover the vast array of plant-based ingredients available to you. Allow your journey to be an evolving process, adapting to your individual needs and preferences.

Seek out a supportive community—whether it be friends, family, or online networks—that shares your passion for plant-based living. Share your experiences, learn from others, and draw inspiration from the collective wisdom of those on similar paths. Surrounding yourself with a positive and encouraging environment can make your journey not only more enjoyable but also more sustainable in the long run.

In conclusion, adopting a plant-based, anti-inflammatory lifestyle is a profound act of self-care. It is an investment in your health, the well-being of the planet, and the interconnectedness of all living things. Embrace this journey with gratitude for the nourishment it provides, celebrate the successes along the way, and approach challenges as opportunities for growth. May your path be filled with vibrant health, joy, and the fulfillment that comes from making choices aligned with your values and the well-being of the world around you. Here's to a lifelong journey to health!